LEGIONNAIRES DISEASE

Ways To Protect Yourself Against Legionnaires Disease At Home

Dr, Tiffany J. Bozeman

CONTENT

INTRODUCTION

CHAPTER ONE

- Introduction To Legionnaires' Disease
- Legionnaires' Disease Signs And Symptoms
- How The Legionnaire's Disease Is Spread
- People at Risk for Legionnaires' Disease

CHAPTER TWO

- Legionella Bacteria Sources In The Household
- Significance Of Water System Maintenance And Cleaning

CHAPTER THREE

- How To Avoid Legionnaires' Disease At Home
- How To Stop Legionella Bacteria From Spreading In Your Home
- Options For Legionella Prevention In Water

CHAPTER FOUR

- How To Act If You Think You May Have Legionnaires' Disease
- What To Do If You Think You May Have Legionnaires' Disease
- Importance Of Quickly Seeking Medical Attention

CHAPTER FIVE

- <u>Factors In Law And Regulation</u>
- <u>Applicable Rules And Recommendations For Preventing Legionnaires' Disease In The Home</u>
- <u>Legal Considerations For Property Owners And Landlords</u>
- <u>Employers' Obligations Regarding Employees' Protection Against Legionnaires' Disease</u>

INTRODUCTION

Legionella is a bacterium that causes Legionnaires' disease, a severe kind of pneumonia. Droplets of contaminated water from sources like air conditioners, hot tubs, and showers may spread this illness when inhaled. For those with low immune systems, in particular, the illness known as legionnaires' may be fatal. The spread of Legionella bacteria in the house may be stopped, however, by following some simple precautions. This book seeks to provide readers with an in-depth manual on how to avoid Legionnaires' illness at home.

CHAPTER ONE

Introduction To Legionnaires' Disease

The bacterium Legionella causes the severe type of pneumonia known as Legionnaires' disease. Legionnaires' disease is most often brought on by the bacterium Legionella , while other Legionella species are also capable of causing the sickness.

The illness was given the moniker "legionnaires' sickness" when it was first discovered in 1976 during an outbreak at an American Legion conference in Philadelphia.

Legionella bacteria may be found in natural water sources including rivers, lakes, and streams, and flourish in warm, wet settings. Air conditioning units, hot tubs, showers, and beautiful fountains are all examples of man-made habitats where the bacterium may be discovered. These surroundings may contain Legionella bacteria, which may become airborne and be breathed, resulting in Legionnaires' illness.

Legionnaires' Disease Signs And Symptoms

Similar to pneumonia symptoms, the signs and symptoms of legionnaires' disease may range from moderate to severe. Legionnaires' illness typically has an incubation period of two to 10 days. Legionnaires' illness often manifests as:

1. A fever
2. A chill
3. Cough
4. Breathing difficulties
5. pains in your muscles
6. headache
7. Weariness
8. A decrease in hunger
9. Dizziness or confusion

Legionnaires' illness, when left untreated, may cause renal and respiratory failure as well as death. Depending on the patient's age and state of health, the death risk for Legionnaires' illness may vary from 5% to 30%.

How The Legionnaire's Disease Is Spread

Legionella bacteria found in water droplets that have gone airborne may cause Legionnaires' illness when inhaled. This may happen in several contexts, such as:

1. Air conditioning systems: In water used in air conditioning systems to chill the air, Legionella bacteria may proliferate. Legionella bacteria may be discharged into the air and ingested by building occupants if the water is not kept clean.

2. Hot tubs and spas: Legionella bacteria may be found in hot tubs and spas often. For Legionella bacteria to flourish, the warm

water and mist that are produced may be the perfect conditions.

3. Showers and faucets: The water used for showers and faucets is a suitable environment for Legionella bacteria to flourish. Legionella bacteria may be discharged into the air if the temperature is not regulated appropriately or the water is not kept clean.

4. Decorative fountains: The Legionella bacteria may also be found in decorative fountains. Nearby individuals may breathe in the created mist.

People at Risk for Legionnaires' Disease

Legionnaires' disease is more likely to affect some demographic groups than others. They comprise:

1. Elderly folks: Over-50s are more likely to get legionnaires' disease than younger ones.

2. Smokers: Smokers have an increased chance of getting Legionnaires' illness.

3. Those with compromised immune systems: Individuals with compromised immune systems are more likely to get Legionnaires' disease, particularly individuals with HIV/AIDS, cancer, or organ transplants.

4. Those who have underlying medical issues: Those who have underlying health issues, such as diabetes or chronic lung illness, are more likely to get Legionnaires' disease.

5. Recent travelers: Recent travelers, particularly those who have gone overseas, may be more susceptible to getting Legionnaires' illness.

6. Persons in certain professions: Due to their exposure to water systems that may contain Legionella bacteria, some professions, such as those in the healthcare industry, plumbing, and maintenance, may have a greater risk of getting Legionnaires' illness.

CHAPTER TWO

Legionella Bacteria Sources In The Household

Legionella bacteria are often found in natural water sources, but they may also be found in artificial water systems in houses and other structures. Showers, faucets, hot water tanks, water heaters, and ornamental fountains are some of these systems. The common sources of Legionella bacteria in the house and their methods of transmission will be covered in this chapter.

Water Heaters And Hot Water Tanks

In the house, Legionella bacteria are often found in hot water tanks and water heaters. The warm water kept in these systems may support the growth of Legionella bacteria. Legionella bacteria may grow and spread if the water is not adequately managed or the temperature is not regulated appropriately. When hot water is utilized for showers or faucets, the germs may subsequently be discharged into the atmosphere.

Faucets And Showers

Moreover, the water that is utilized for showers and faucets may contain Legionella bacteria. Legionella bacteria may grow and spread if the water is not adequately managed or the temperature is not regulated appropriately. As the water is consumed, the germs may subsequently be discharged into the atmosphere.

Fountains With Ornaments

Legionella bacteria may also be found in decorative fountains. Anyone nearby may breathe in the produced mist and get Legionnaires' disease. To stop the development and spread of Legionella bacteria, beautiful fountains must be regularly maintained and cleaned.

Legionella bacteria may also be found in air conditioning units. The water that air conditioning systems utilize to chill the air may support the growth of Legionella bacteria. Legionella bacteria may be discharged into the air and breathed by individuals in the building if the water is not adequately kept.

Significance Of Water System Maintenance And Cleaning

To stop the development and spread of Legionella bacteria, water systems in the house must be properly maintained and cleaned. To avoid the accumulation of silt that might contain the Legionella bacteria, this includes:

1. Routinely emptying hot water tanks and water heaters.

2. To stop the development of Legionella bacteria, hot water tanks, and water heaters should be set to a temperature of at least 140°F.

3. Routinely sanitizing and cleaning faucets and showerheads to stop the development and spread of Legionella bacteria.

4. Doing routine cleaning and disinfection of ornamental fountains to stop Legionella bacteria development and spread.

5. Doing routine cleaning and disinfection of air conditioning units to stop Legionella bacteria from growing and spreading.

It is crucial to be aware of the signs of Legionnaires' illness and seek medical assistance if required, in addition to performing regular maintenance and cleaning. Elderly individuals, smokers, and those with compromised immune systems are at a greater risk of developing Legionnaires' illness and should take additional steps to avoid coming into contact with Legionella bacteria.

Water systems in the house, such as hot water tanks, water heaters, showers, faucets, and ornamental fountains, may harbor Legionella bacteria. To stop the development and spread of the Legionella bacteria and lower the risk of Legionnaires' illness, these systems must be properly maintained and cleaned.

CHAPTER THREE

How To Avoid Legionnaires' Disease At Home

To lower the danger of Legionnaires' illness, it is crucial to stop the spread of Legionella bacteria within the house. In this chapter, we will go through ways to stop the spread of Legionella bacteria in the house, the significance of maintaining a consistent water system temperature, and several water treatment solutions.

How To Stop Legionella Bacteria From Spreading In Your Home

1. Regular maintenance and cleaning of water systems: To stop the development and spread of Legionella bacteria, regular maintenance, and cleaning of water systems in the house are crucial. This includes cleaning and sanitizing showerheads, faucets, and ornamental fountains in addition to draining out hot water tanks and water heaters.

2. Temperature control: It's essential to keep water systems at the right temperature to stop the development of Legionella bacteria. To stop the formation of the Legionella bacteria, hot water tanks, and water heaters should be set at a minimum temperature of 140°F. Legionella bacteria shouldn't be allowed to develop in cold

water, which should be maintained below 68°F.

3. Remove stagnant water as much as possible: Legionella bacteria thrive in stagnant water. Hence, it's crucial to reduce standing water in the house by using the taps and showers often and avoiding extended periods of inactivity.

4. Air conditioning systems: To stop the development and spread of Legionella bacteria, air conditioning systems should be constantly maintained and cleaned.

Controlling temperature is crucial in water systems.

Controlling the temperature is essential for avoiding the development of Legionella bacteria. To stop the formation of Legionella bacteria, hot water tanks, and water heaters should be set at a minimum temperature of 140°F. Legionella bacteria shouldn't be allowed to develop in cold water, which should be maintained below 68°F. The danger of Legionnaires' illness is decreased by keeping water systems at the right temperature, which also hinders the development of the bacterium Legionella.

Options For Legionella Prevention In Water

To stop Legionella bacteria from multiplying and spreading, a variety of water treatment solutions are available. They consist of:

1. Chlorine: To eliminate Legionella bacteria, chlorine is a frequent water treatment technique. To guarantee that chlorine is efficient in destroying germs, it is crucial to utilize the right concentration.

2. Copper-silver ionization: This method of water purification releases copper and silver ions into the water by the use of electrodes. These ions can eliminate Legionella bacteria thanks to their antibacterial characteristics.

3. Ultraviolet light: By causing Genetic damage to Legionella bacteria, ultraviolet light may be utilized to destroy them. This is a good Legionella preventative water treatment solution.

4. Hyperchlorination: To eradicate the Legionella bacteria, hyperchlorination requires raising the chlorine content in water systems. This approach for water treatment is efficient, but to guarantee that it is done properly, it should only be used by skilled specialists.

To lower the danger of Legionnaires' illness, it is crucial to stop the spread of Legionella bacteria within the house. To stop the development and spread of Legionella bacteria, it's crucial to maintain water systems regularly, manage the temperature, eliminate standing water, and regularly clean and disinfect air conditioning systems. Legionella bacteria may also be prevented from growing and dispersing by using water treatment techniques including chlorine, copper-silver ionization, ultraviolet radiation, and hyperchlorination.

CHAPTER FOUR

How To Act If You Think You May Have Legionnaires' Disease

The deadly sickness known as legionnaires' disease needs immediate medical intervention. In this chapter, we'll go over what to do if you think you could have Legionnaires' disease, why it's crucial to get medical help right away, and how to report possible instances.

What To Do If You Think You May Have Legionnaires' Disease

The following actions should be performed if you believe you or someone in your household has Legionnaires' disease:

1. Get urgent medical treatment: The first step is to seek emergency medical attention. If the Legionnaires' illness is not treated right away, it may be fatal. It's critical to get medical assistance as quickly as possible since the symptoms of Legionnaires' disease might resemble those of other respiratory disorders, such as pneumonia.

2. Tell your physician: Let your physician know that you think you may have Legionnaires' disease. To confirm the

diagnosis and choose the best course of action, your doctor will probably prescribe tests.

3. Determine the bacteria's source: If you have been diagnosed with Legionnaires' illness, it's critical to determine the bacteria's source. This may aid in limiting the bacteria's ability to infect others and averting further outbreaks.

4. Adhere to the recommended course of action: Antibiotics are often used to treat legionnaires' illnesses. It's crucial to adhere to the recommended course of therapy and take all drugs as prescribed.

Importance Of Quickly Seeking Medical Attention

If you have any suspicions about Legionnaires' disease, you must get medical help right once. If the Legionnaires' illness is not treated right away, it may be fatal. Early detection and intervention may lessen problems and increase the likelihood of a complete recovery.

Reporting Potential Legionnaires' Disease Cases

It's crucial to report suspected instances of Legionnaires' illness to stop the bacteria's spread and find probable infection sources. All suspected instances of Legionnaires' disease should be reported to the local health authority, which will then investigate to determine the source of the bacterium and take the necessary precautions to stop any more illnesses.

The deadly sickness known as legionnaires' disease needs immediate medical intervention. It is crucial to seek medical assistance right once, tell your doctor that you think you may have Legionnaires' disease, locate the source of the bacteria, and adhere to the recommended treatment schedule. It's crucial to report suspected instances of Legionnaires' illness to stop the bacteria's spread and find probable infection sources. By adopting these actions, we may contribute to the prevention of the Legionnaires' illness and safeguard our health and the health and safety of those around us.

CHAPTER FIVE

Factors In Law And Regulation

The deadly infection known as legionnaires' disease may have wide-ranging legal and regulatory repercussions. In this chapter, we'll talk about the laws that apply to preventing Legionnaires' disease in the house, the legal obligations of property owners and landlords, and the obligations of employers to safeguard their employees from Legionnaires' disease.

Applicable Rules And Recommendations For Preventing Legionnaires' Disease In The Home

The prevention of Legionnaires' disease in the home is governed by several laws and rules. Among the important rules and directives are:

1. Occupational Safety and Health Administration (OSHA) Recommendations: OSHA has produced recommendations for workplace prevention of Legionnaires' disease. These suggestions cover control strategies to stop Legionella bacteria development in water systems as well as water management initiatives.

2. Recommendations created by the Centers for Disease Control and Prevention (CDC) for the prevention of Legionnaires' disease in healthcare institutions. These suggestions include water management, disinfection, and water system maintenance.

3. ASHRAE Standards of the American Society of Heating, Refrigerating, and Air-Conditioning Engineers: Standards for preventing Legionnaires' disease in structures have been set by ASHRAE. Recommendations for temperature control, water system disinfection, and water management strategies are all included in these standards.

Legal Considerations For Property Owners And Landlords:

It is required by law for landlords and property owners to provide their tenants with safe, livable dwellings. It is possible to face legal repercussions for failing to take the necessary precautions to avoid Legionnaires' disease. Among the legal issues that landlords and property owners should think about are:

1. Responsibility to Keep Safe Housing: Landlords have a responsibility to keep their tenants in safe homes. This entails taking the proper precautions to avoid contracting the Legionnaires' illness, such as keeping water systems clean and maintained.

2. Responsibility to Alert Tenants to Risks: Landlords are responsible for alerting renters to recognized dangers, such as the presence of Legionella bacteria in water systems.

3. Negligence Liability: If a landlord neglects to take reasonable precautions to avoid Legionnaires' disease and a tenant contracts the illness as a consequence, the landlord may be held accountable for negligence.

Employers' Obligations Regarding Employees' Protection Against Legionnaires' Disease

Employers have to ensure that workers are working in a safe environment. This involves taking the necessary precautions to avoid Legionnaires' disease at work. Employers have a responsibility to take the following actions to safeguard employees against Legionnaires' disease:

1. Creating a Water Management Program: To stop Legionella bacteria from growing in water systems, employers should create a water management program. This program needs to include routine cleaning, disinfection, and supervision of water systems.

2. Teaching Employees: Companies must inform staff members of the dangers of Legionnaires' disease and the best ways to avoid it. This may include instructing how to properly clean and disinfect water systems.

3. Supplying Personal Protective Equipment (PPE): Companies should provide personnel who could be exposed to Legionella germs the proper PPE, such as respirators.

The deadly infection known as legionnaires' disease may have wide-ranging legal and regulatory repercussions. If the right steps are not taken to avoid Legionnaires' disease, landlords and property owners may be held accountable for carelessness. They are legally obligated to provide safe housing for their tenants. Businesses must create a water management program, inform staff members of the dangers of Legionnaires' disease, and supply the necessary equipment to ensure that workers operate in a safe environment. We can safeguard our health and the health and safety of people around us by taking these steps to help stop the spread of Legionnaires' disease.

www.ingramcontent.com/pod-product-compliance
Lightning Source LLC
Chambersburg PA
CBHW050753250726
48662CB00005B/2197